BodyDesigns
Two-Week Detox Plan
Lose Weight and Get Healthy

Mary Sabat MS, RDN, LD

The recommendations in this book are not meant to replace the advice given to you by your physician. The information given to you in this book is designed to help you make important decisions about your health, lose weight and get healthy. If you take medications or have a medical illness in which a physician is following you please do not replace this information with that of your doctor. Always consult a physician before beginning any diet or detox plan. The information in this book is not intended for pregnant or nursing women. The author disclaims any liability directly or indirectly from any use of the material in this book by any person.

Mention of specific products or companies, or authorities in this book does not imply endorsement by the author nor does it imply that such companies or authorities endorse this book or author.

Table of Contents

Introduction

"Let food be thy medicine and medicine be thy food."
– Hippocrates

If you are reading this, then you have already made a commitment to take charge of your health. What you have in your hands is not just a powerful two-week Detox Plan to lose weight, but a strong beginning to a lifetime of optimal wellness. This book will give you the tools you need to commit to and take charge of your health. I'm excited to lead you through this journey down the path to health and vitality.

For over 20 years, I have helped people lose weight and get well. I was surprised to find out that what was believed to be common knowledge about nutrition and health and what I was taught in school many years ago is not what I know to be true today. All of the textbooks and classrooms in the world simply cannot substitute for the years of experience I've gained by working with real people on a daily basis. My knowledge base was formed by experiencing firsthand - what works and what doesn't work when it comes to weight loss and health.

Like most people, you may be solely focused on weight loss and that's great! BodyDesigns Two-Week Detox Plan is focused on losing weight however, weight loss goes hand-in-hand with health. All of the things that make you fat are the things that make you sick. If you were honest, many of you would admit that you have other health symptoms, besides

1

body fat that bother you. You are lucky if, with your current excess weight, you still haven't experienced any other difficulty or symptoms of dwindling health. Now is the time to lose that excess fat to prevent your body from getting sick! My unique and detailed Detox Plan is designed to let you lose those unwanted pounds and lead you to optimal wellness at the same time.

My hope for you in reading this book is that you embark on this plan with the idea that food is your medicine. When we let our food nourish and heal our bodies and eliminate the foods causing inflammation and disease we will see the weight come off easily as we begin to feel great and enjoy optimal health and wellness.

Wishing you a lifetime of good health.

– Mary

Chapter 1: Understanding the Purpose of Detoxification

"Take care of your body. It's the only place you have to live."
– Jim Rohn

This Detox Plan will both add food to and remove food from your diet. It eliminates gluten, dairy, sugar and processed foods that may prevent you from losing weight and make you sick, while adding nourishing foods that you need to make your body well and promote fat burn. In spite of hard work, many people cannot lose weight because their intestinal tracts or "guts" are unhealthy and their livers are not functioning properly. The systems meant to detoxify one's body are malfunctioning. The gut and the liver are two of our bodies' primary detoxification systems and both must be healthy in order to facilitate weight loss. Fortunately, in the same way that excess weight and illness create a negative feedback loop, detoxification and weight loss strengthen each other and create a positive momentum toward increased good health.

Many people today suffer from dysbiosis, which is an overgrowth of bad bacteria in the intestinal lining. This disruption in the normal gut ecosystem leads to a "leaky gut". A "leaky gut" allows toxins and substances into the body causing an array of problems including inflammation, autoimmune reactions, and allergies. Inflammation in the body causes disease and also prevents your body from losing weight. The Detox Plan will immediately start healing your gut by removing the foods that may be causing inflammation and the toxins that make it unhealthy. The diet adds nourishing foods that enable good bacteria to flourish in your system. Since the gut is responsible for 70% of our body's immune function, a healthy gut means a healthy body.

The second most important organ in our body that could affect our health is the liver. The liver must be able to effectively break down fats and eliminate toxins. Many people with excess belly fat around the middle also have a fatty liver. Fatty liver must be reversed so that the liver can do its job. If we don't reverse this problem, weight loss will be extremely difficult if not impossible.

The morning lemon water and spirulina in your shake are key to helping you detox your liver and your gut. The Detox Soup is taken once a day and is full of natural detoxifying ingredients that will help to heal not only the liver, but the intestinal tract as well. In addition, the high fiber intake in the plan allows for the beneficial bacteria in the gut to grow and populate for optimal immunity and health. Healthy fats are key as they aid in reducing inflammation and help keep you satisfied as they replace the missing calories that your body has been getting from unhealthy amounts of carbohydrates.

*"For me the detox was an eye opening experience.
I lost 12 lbs., eliminated my reflux and IBS symptoms and
learned that I was intolerant to gluten. In addition, my chronic
pain issues are almost entirely gone. It was easy to follow and
it will forever change the way I eat."*

– Jessica T., Delaware

Chapter 2:
The Truth Behind the
Standard American Diet
(SAD)

"Eating crappy food isn't a reward -- it's a punishment."
– Drew Carey

The Standard American Diet, also known as S.A.D. is used to describe the typical dietary patterns of Americans. Most Americans are eating a high percentage of calories from sugar, grains, processed foods and fake or "Frankenfoods". "Frankenfoods" are made by food manufacturers who mix food and chemicals to create certain tastes and flavors that mimic real food. The high sugar and toxin load of this typical American diet sets us up for obesity and disease.

The S.A.D. is rich in sugar and unhealthy fats and deficient in healthy fats. Healthy fats are needed for nearly every aspect of bodily functions, including immunity, brain health, gut health, and hormone regulation. Our ancestors did not eat this way. In fact, up until the 1950's our food supply was much different. Back in 1955 a researcher by the name of Keys offered a hypothesis at the World Health Organization in Geneva. Keys theory was that dietary fat raised cholesterol, subsequently increasing the risk of heart disease. His research did not take into account many other factors, one of which was a high sugar diet. Based on this false assumption, the food industry responded by producing vast amounts of low fat foods, which were supposed to help people lose weight and prevent heart disease. Unfortunately, the fat that was removed from these foods was replaced with large amounts of sugar and chemicals. Sadly, as our foods increased in sugar and chemicals, so did the rate of obesity and heart disease. In fact, many health problems increased as a direct result of this new Standard American Diet (S.A.D.) including diabetes, hypertension, depression, autoimmune diseases, allergies, autism, ADD, fatigue, mood disorders and the list goes on.

Many people still believe that all fat is bad for us, when in reality, health problems, such as the heart disease epidemic, are far more closely related to trans fats (fake fat created by the food industry) and sugar and not natural healthy fats that nature intended for us to eat.

Of course animal fat is where toxins are stored so the leanest cuts of poultry and beef are usually best to avoid the dangers of hidden toxins and chemicals but saturated fats are not the culprit! It's time to make a huge change and stop being afraid of adding fat to our diet. The Detox Plan gets you started eating more healthy fats in place of the missing sugar and grains and this change will be a main factor in your lifelong success at not only keeping weight off but maintaining good health.

Depriving the body of the nutrients it needs by eating a highly processed diet can be equally as bad. The lack of healthy fats in the S.A.D. causes widespread deficiency of vitamin D, which is crucial in fighting cancer and protecting our bones and many other vital organs in the body. Highly processed foods are deficient in essential vitamins, minerals and phytonutrients, which can be linked to just about any disease state or ailment such as fatigue, allergies, hypo-thyroidism, asthma, cancer and autoimmune diseases.

The average American consumes 130 lbs. of sugar every year. Sugar is an addictive substance. Studies have shown that, for some, it can be as addictive as alcohol or cocaine. Many people scoff at the idea of an obese person not being able to control a craving for sugar however, based on science and research, we now know that sugar is physically addicting.

Remember also that all carbohydrates turn to sugar in the body. So, whether it comes from a gluten free piece of bread or a piece of cotton candy, your body will break it down to sugar and respond in the same way producing insulin which stores fat. However, carbohydrates from most vegetables (non-starchy) will not react the same way because of the high fiber content that slows down the absorption of sugar. Therefore vegetables won't cause high spikes in insulin and at the same time are loading our bodies with nourishment that keeps us well.

The S.A.D is also full of chemicals like M.S.G. that make your body crave more of the very food that you should not be eating. Many people today are truly addicted to fast food. It's no mistake that when you eat these foods you crave them even more. The manufacturing companies know what to put in the food to make you come back again and again and these chemicals and substances can make you fat and sick!

One of the important purposes of this Detox Plan is to completely eliminate foods that may be causing inflammation and weight gain. Once you rid yourself of these addictive foods, you will stop craving them… I promise! With just a few days worth of commitment and determination, this Detox Plan will completely change your health and well-being. By the end of the two weeks, your body will be craving only real food. Food that will feed your body with what it needs to be healthy and, at the same time, lose weight.

"Prior to the Detox Plan I was craving sweets and processed foods. After the first few days all my food cravings completely went away and I felt more in control of myself. I also had good energy, my anxiety disappeared and I was not hungry at all. My IBS symptoms have disappeared and I no longer have gas, bloating or general gastric irritation. I lost 9 lbs. on the detox and continued to lose to a total of 26 lbs. I feel great and highly recommend this detox plan to everyone.
– Lynn L., Georgia

Chapter 3:
The Hormones Behind Your Weight

"Laughter is the best medicine – unless you're diabetic, then insulin comes pretty high up on the list."

– Jasper Carrott

Hormones are substances in the body that control and regulate bodily functions such as digestion, metabolism, growth, reproduction, and mood. Controlling our weight comes down to being able to control our hormones. I find that once people understand the concept of how these weight related hormones work, they are able to lose weight and keep it off for good.

The Detox Plan is about balancing four critical hormones that are crucial for weight loss to take place. This plan is formulated to get these hormones working FOR you instead of AGAINST you for optimal weight loss. First, you must balance insulin and glucagon which act as a kind of hormonal "yin and yang". Insulin is the hormone that affects fat storage while glucagon affects the breakdown of fat. The body cannot simultaneously have high levels of insulin and glucagon. The pancreas secretes insulin in response to rising glucose (sugar) levels in the blood while secreting glucagon when the glucose levels fall. As the insulin levels rise, the body stores more fat. Thus, the more sugar you consume the higher your insulin levels rise. Over eating, especially from carbohydrate rich foods, lead to more glucose, which leads to an increase in stored fat, typically around our abdominal region. Worse, this type of stored fat becomes resistant to insulin requiring the pancreas to produce even more insulin. So the cycle begins: the fatter we get the sicker we get and the sicker we get the fatter we get.

High insulin levels in the body will eventually lead to Type 2 diabetes. In fact, some doctors are now testing for insulin levels as an early predictor of diabetes. Diabesity is a term used to describe a range from a mild insulin resistance to full blown diabetes. It's the high insulin levels that begin the vicious cycle of storing fat, increasing hunger, and producing inflammation, which in turn all lead to disease. The more we feed into this cycle of spiking high insulin levels the more we become fat and sick. Your doctor may not diagnose you with diabetes but high insulin levels begin the disease process long before your doctor sees it in your blood work.

The good news is that once you know how to stop that chain reaction you are one step closer to significantly improving your health and losing weight. So where does the sugar in our body come from? Easy: from carbohydrates. Carbohydrates, both the "good" ones and the "bad" ones, all turn into sugar in the body. Therefore, to control sugar intake, you must control carbohydrate intake. The Two-Week Detox Plan teaches you how to control the quantity of carbohydrate intake and how to eat the right carbohydrates and combine foods the right way to significantly limit your body's insulin response.

Keep in mind you are eliminating gluten for gut health as well as for the effect these grains have on insulin levels. Gluten is a protein found in certain grains such as wheat, rye and barley. For some people gluten, like dairy, may be causing inflammation and preventing them from being able to lose weight. Once the detox is over, you can replace small amounts of gluten in the diet as a trial to see if you get negative symptoms. However, you don't want to go back to the S.A.D., which is high in processed sugar and carbohydrates. Many processed gluten free products are also carbohydrate rich foods that will spike insulin levels too high if eaten too frequently, in large amounts or without the proper food combinations.

The other two hormones that must be considered for weight loss are leptin and ghrelin. Leptin and ghrelin have been called the "hunger hormones" because they are directly involved in appetite control. Leptin helps control appetite by suppressing food intake, letting our bodies know that we are satiated. Ghrelin has the opposite effect by making us so hungry that we can't feel full. Ghrelin has been nicknamed the "pig out" hormone because as levels rise too high, appetite can't be tamed and overeating occurs.

Leptin increases during sleep telling the brain that it has enough energy. People who don't sleep well or sleep enough will have decreased levels of leptin and will feel hungry all day long. On the other hand, people who don't sleep enough produce too much ghrelin. Ghrelin tells the brain that it needs energy and needs to eat. Ghrelin also increases when you go too long without food. People who skip meals or go longer then 4 hours without a meal or snack will have higher levels of ghrelin and will have a harder time regulating their food intake.

So the Detox Plan controls ghrelin by having you eat several meals and snacks throughout the day. Never wait more then 4 hours between meals and snacks as the hungrier you get the harder it will be to stick to the plan. Having a good sleep routine also controls leptin and ghrelin. Be sure to get at least 7-9 hours of sleep every night. Increase your exercise level for better sleep but don't exercise within 3 hours of bedtime. Lastly, although you wouldn't do this on the detox plan, for future purposes don't ingest caffeine or alcohol too close to bedtime as it can disrupt normal sleep patterns.

"I just completed Mary's two-week detox and I feel amazing. I lost 9.5 lbs. pounds. Almost 10 lbs. in two weeks is amazing! But the best part is I didn't feel hungry or deprived while detoxing, and I was able to stick with it while traveling and eating out. My clothes fit again and the detox program launched me into a healthier, cleaner lifestyle. Thanks Mary!"
– Liz D., Georgia

Chapter 4:
What to Expect

"The secret to getting ahead is getting started."
– Mark Twain

During the first few days on the Detox Plan, you may feel tired or have a slight headache as your body adjusts to the lower carbohydrate level and flushes out the toxins that have been keeping you from losing weight. Most people feel more energy and begin to feel great by day 3 as their bodies have adjusted and are beginning to burn fat.

During the detox, if you should feel hungry, I advise you to add more healthy fats and some vegetables that are allowed on the Detox Plan. Protein should be kept to the recommended portion sizes for your body weight. Be sure to drink plenty of water to allow your body to get rid of the toxins as you burn off fat.

People report losing anywhere from 5 to 13 pounds on this plan with an average weight loss of 8 lbs. The amount you lose seems to be proportionate not only to your starting weight but also to your intolerance to dairy or gluten. Dairy or gluten intolerant people with very little to lose may lose 10 pounds while those who are not intolerant to gluten or diary might lose less. Either way everyone reports positive effects on their health such as decreased or elimination of inflammation, no longer craving sweets, sleeping better and having more energy.

Once you finish the Detox Plan, gluten and dairy are reintroduced one at a time so that you can determine if either of these has been a culprit in your weight or health issues. Most people never go back to at least one of these as they realize right away how they feel once they add one back.

After following The Two-Week Detox Plan for 14 days, be sure to consider a Personalized Diet Plan. For information about a diet plan that can help you transition to your new lifestyle to continue losing weight or for weight maintenance go to BodyDesignsbyMary.com.

Chapter 5:
Determining Portion Size

"Life itself is the proper binge."

– Julia Child

Please note that portions of protein and the number of afternoon snacks vary depending upon your current weight. If you have 75 pounds or less to lose, stick with the lower range of protein listed such as 3 ounces of chicken or 6 ounces of tofu. For example, a man or woman wishing to lose 45 pounds might have 3 ounces of chicken at a meal. A man or women wishing to lose 75 pounds or more would be able to have 4 ounces of chicken at a meal. For the afternoon snack, people needing to lose less then 75 lbs. may have 1 snack and people needing to lose more then 75 lbs. may have 2 snacks.

The morning snack should be soup and the afternoon snack should be from the list as suggested. The evening snack is a Grain Free Cake or you may switch it with the Detox Soup or choose from the afternoon snack list.

The evening snack is optional but please don't skip all of your snacks as eating throughout the day is important for hormonal balance.

At the end of the day, portion control is important. Eating the right food is key, but we can't over eat even the healthiest foods and expect to lose weight. Beware of any diet plan that suggests unlimited calories throughout the day. The bottom line is we must have a calorie deficit to achieve weight loss, unless we are in a state of starvation with very little carbohydrate intake at all, which is not what this plan is proposing.

"I went on Mary's detox plan and lost 8 lbs. in just two weeks! My digestion has never felt better as I am now regular and no longer struggle with any gastrointestinal issues. I have continued to work with Mary on a personal diet plan and I continue to lose weight. The detox plan worked for me and it was so easy to follow. It reprogrammed the way I think about eating and made it very easy to transition into the lifestyle diet plan that Mary prepared for me."

– Lucie S., Georgia

Chapter 6:
Getting Prepared
for Success

*"Planning is bringing the future into the present
so that you can do something about it now."*
— Alan Lakein

Make sure you are prepared for the detox both mentally and physically. Think ahead to be sure your schedule for the two weeks doesn't interfere with the diet. You can successfully stick to this diet even while traveling or eating out with a little planning but too many events during the two weeks may make it tough. Next, make sure you do your grocery shopping and prepare your foods in advance so you are ready to start on day one.

You are allowed to drink one cup of organic coffee daily. If you drink a lot of coffee, start to slowly decrease intake over the few days prior to the detox so the shock to your system is not so sudden. Caffeine withdrawal can cause bad headaches. I recommend you use Teeccino (an herbal coffee substitute) in place of half of your regular coffee in each cup until you have it down to 1 cup of coffee daily. Make sure you are only using organic coffee or tea. Coffee and tea crops are highly sprayed with pesticides and non-organic coffee or tea will disrupt your detox process.

Make the Detox Soup recipe found in the Recipe section of this book and freeze half of it for the second week. The recipe makes a lot of soup. Once the kale is added to the pot it will become very thick. Add several cups of water to thin out the soup to a consistency of your liking. Feel free to spice up the soup if you don't find it tasty enough, although most people do not need additional seasonings.

Pre package your snacks such as nuts into portion sizes that you can grab and take with you to work or on the go. Having fresh vegetables cleaned and cut up will save you time and help keep you on track when you are busy. If you like hummus, prepare a batch of Cauliflower Hummus and keep it in the refrigerator in 1/2-cup containers. Many people find that the hummus makes a delicious salad dressing too.

Prepare your protein and have it ready in 3-4 ounce portions (portions depend on your size, please read Chapter 5: Determining Portion Size). Plan to keep several days worth of grilled chicken, hard-boiled eggs, etc. in the refrigerator to make it easier to stay on the plan.

The Shopping List can be found in Appendix 2. Make a copy of the shopping list so that you can check off what you need or want to buy and write in your vegetables of choice for the week. Keep in mind that the list is a guideline for things you may want to purchase, but not all the items are necessary. Plan your meals and snacks first then make the list. Appendix 3 is also found at the end of the book and has guidelines to assist you on where to buy some items.

Pick your start date and let's begin getting this weight off and getting your health back!

"I did Mary's Detox Plan in June and lost 8 lbs. After a few days I developed a headache and I think it was from my body withdrawing from sugar and toxic foods that I no longer eat. After the initial week I noticed the swelling under my kneecap that has plagued me for years was diminished. I no longer have the rumbling gut syndrome that I had before eliminating dairy and gluten. My cravings for sweets and carbohydrates were gone by the 4th day. I have kept my weight off and continued to lose to a total of 25 lbs. following Mary's personal diet plan that she did for me. It was such an easy transition from the detox to my new lifestyle. I love how I eat and I love how I feel as the detox changed my eating habits forever."
–Janet T. Georgia

Chapter 7:
Quick Overview
of the Plan

Upon rising – 12 ounces of Lemon water

Breakfast – Vegan shake

1 cup Organic Coffee or Tea is optional

Snack- 1 cup Detox soup (or save it for later)

Lunch

- 1 serving of protein (portion depends on body weight and protein source)
- Choose several vegetables from the Unlimited Vegetable List
- Choose 1 - 2 healthy fats from Healthy Fats List
- Optional – 1 small sweet potato, ½ cup quinoa, ½ cup brown rice
- Salad with organic greens recommended

Snack – choose 1 or 2 (depends on body weight) from list

Dinner

- 1 serving protein (portion depends on body weight and protein source)
- Choose several vegetables from the Unlimited Vegetable List
- Choose 1- 2 healthy fats from Healthy Fats List
- Salad with organic greens recommended

Snack – Grain Free Quick Cake or snack from afternoon list

Drink lots of water to remove toxins and stay hydrated

Exercise – sweating helps remove toxins from your body

Sleep 7-8 hours each night to balance hormones

Chapter 8: Detailed Instructions

"To get rich never risk your health.
For it is the truth that Health is the Wealth of Wealth."
— Richard Baker

On the first day of the detox, be sure to weigh yourself first thing in the morning. If you wish you can also take some starting measurements too.

Lemon Water

Start each day with lemon water on an empty stomach.

- *Lemon Water*
- 12 oz. lukewarm water
- 2 T lemon juice (about ½ of a lemon)

Warm lemon water has been used since ancient times as a natural remedy for digestive problems. Lemons will support your detox by normalizing your digestive enzymes, help to move roughage through the body and reduce bloating. In addition lemons will activate the liver to release toxins necessary for your body to begin breaking down fats.

Keep it by your bathroom sink and drink it down first thing in the morning so it's at room temperature or heat it to lukewarm and add lemon. Feel free to add lemon to your water all day also. A little stevia can be added to make lemonade.

Organic Coffee or Tea (Optional)

One cup of organic coffee or tea is allowed. Unusual on a detox, but I want you to stick with this so there are a few things allowed that are different from your typical detox. The coffee or tea must be organic because both are highly sprayed crops and the pesticides are going to make it harder for your liver to detox. You may add unsweetened almond, cashew or coconut milk along with stevia to the coffee or tea. Stevia must be a natural leaf stevia (see recommendations below). You can drink organic herbal tea or Teeccino herbal coffee substitute as you desire throughout the day. Note that when you use the almond, cashew or coconut milk in your beverage, be sure it does not contain any carrageenan. Carrageenan is disruptive and possibly carcinogenic to the gut.

Breakfast Shake

Your breakfast shake will be made using a vegan protein powder. I recommend Sunwarrior Raw Blend because it's very clean and tastes great. Other acceptable choices include Garden of Life Raw or Plant Fusion. You can get a flavor like chocolate or vanilla. If you wish to use an alternative vegan shake be sure it is not sweetened with sugar. Acceptable sweeteners that will not raise insulin levels are stevia or Lou Han (Monk Fruit). Lo Han is a natural sweetener that has been used in China for centuries. It comes from the Lo Han fruit and does not appear to affect blood sugar levels. It is considered to be a safe, natural sweetener like stevia and may be used in your plan. These protein powders can be found at a good health food store such as The Vitamin Shoppe or online. After the shopping list you will find suggestions for where to find certain items including the shakes.

The morning shake can be made in a regular blender then you can take it with you in a travel container if desired. The chia seeds need to be soaked in the milk for at least 15 minutes before you make the shake. I recommend pouring the milk in the blender the night before and adding your chia seeds so they are soaked and ready when you want to make the shake.

- 1 scoop Vegan protein powder
- 1 T chia seeds (soaked in the milk for 15-20 minutes)
- 12 ounces unsweetened vanilla or plain almond, cashew or coconut milk
- 1 tsp. organic spirulina powder *or greens (see below)
- ½ banana or ¼ avocado (avocado is a lower sugar option)
- ½ cup organic berries (or you can save them for later in the day)
- Optional for clients over 200 lbs. – add 1 T almond butter or coconut oil

*please read below regarding possible contraindications for using spirulina.

What is Spirulina and Should You Include It?

Spirulina is blue green algae that is rich in chlorophyll and many other life giving nutrients. Spirulina continues the detox process by ridding the body of heavy metals and toxins. It has been labeled a "super food" for its ability to increase immunity, inhibit allergic reactions, treat anemia, cleanse the blood, provide essential amino acids, B vitamins, beneficial bacteria, trace minerals and more, reduce inflammation and even assist in weight loss.

Be sure to buy an organic spirulina to ensure it is not a contaminated source. Only pure, clean sources of spirulina are beneficial and cheap sources may be contaminated and do more harm then good.

In rare cases spirulina may be contraindicated. If you are allergic to seafood, shellfish or iodine do not use it as it may cause a reaction. People being treated with any type of medication for an autoimmune disease should consult their physician before taking spirulina. Anyone with the metabolic condition known as phenylketonuria must also avoid spirulina as they will not be able to break down the amino acid found in the algae. If you should experience severe detoxification symptoms such as sleepiness, itchy skin, excessive gas or other unpleasant symptoms decrease your dose. Pregnant and lactating women should also avoid spirulina as detoxification during this time is not recommended.

Replacing Spirulina in the Shake with Greens

If you fall into any of the categories above you will need to avoid the spirulina and can replace it with 2 cups of organic kale or power greens. If you have a high-speed blender you will be able to blend the greens right into your shake. If you can't blend them into your shake you can lightly sauté the greens and eat them on the side each morning.

What are Chia Seeds?

Chia seeds come from a plant native to Mexico and Guatemala and have long been an important food crop in those countries. In 1991, Wayne Coates began researching the seeds and has since become a huge advocate for their health benefits. Unlike flaxseeds, chia seeds can be eaten whole so no grinding is required.

Chia seeds are also considered a super food as they are full of nourishing nutrients. Chia seeds are an excellent source of omega 3 and 6 fatty acids. Omega 3 fatty acids are powerful anti-inflammatories. The seeds contain soluble and insoluble fiber that help clean out the digestive tract, eliminating toxins. Chia seeds help stabilize blood sugar and bind cholesterol to take it out of the body. In addition, the seeds pack a nutritional punch containing calcium, phosphorus, manganese, and amino acids.

One of the best properties of chia seeds is their ability to soak up water and become a thickening agent. Soaking the seeds for 15-20 minutes creates a gel that is an excellent ingredient in your morning shake or Chia Seed Milkshake snack. Chia seeds can be used in recipes as an egg substitute by combining 1 T chia seeds with 3 T water for every egg being replaced. Enjoy chia seeds on salads or in a variety of recipes as an easy way to add this super food to your diet.

Snack: Detox Soup

This Detox Soup is a recipe that was modified starting with some basics from Dr. Oz's Vegetable Broth. The soup is very tasty and filling and full of vegetables that aid in cleaning out your system and nourishing your body. The 1-cup portion of this soup will fill you up. Try having it as a late morning snack however it is optional to have at any time during the day or with a meal.

Lunch

1. Include 3-4* ounces of organic poultry, wild caught salmon, sardines, or grass-fed beef, 2-3*organic eggs, 6-8* ounces organic tofu, or 3-4* ounces organic tempeh
2. Include vegetables as a side dish from the Unlimited Vegetable List
3. Optional but recommended– large organic greens salad

4. Include 1 -2 healthy fats either mixed into your protein, added on the salad, cooked into the meal or on the side of your plate.

Healthy Fat choices:

- ¼ avocado
- ½ T coconut oil
- ½T olive oil
- 1/2-cup Cauliflower Hummus (recipe below)
- 1/8-cup raw seeds (pumpkin or sunflower)
- 14 raw walnut halves
- 20 raw almonds
- Optional if needed – 1 small sweet potato, ½ cup cooked quinoa, or ½ cup brown rice

Sample Lunch:

- 3 ounces of grilled chicken with 1/4 avocado on top
- 2 cups organic baby greens with 1 T Bragg's Sesame Ginger Dressing, tomatoes, cucumbers and onions
- 1 small sweet potato with stevia and cinnamon

Snack (choose 1-2)*

- 1/2 cup Cauliflower Hummus with cut up vegetables
- 1/2 avocado or 1/4-cup guacamole with cut up vegetables
- 40 pistachios
- 25 almonds

- 14 walnut halves
- ¼ cup raw mixed nuts
- 1 T organic almond butter
- 1 T organic cashew butter
- Chia Seed Milkshake

Dinner

1. Include 3-4* ounces of organic poultry, wild caught salmon, sardines, or grass-fed beef, 2-3*organic eggs, 6-8* ounces organic tofu, or 3-4* ounces organic tempeh
2. Include vegetables as a side dish from the Unlimited Vegetable List
3. Optional but recommended– large organic greens salad
4. Include 1 -2 healthy fats either mixed into your protein, added on the salad, cooked into the meal or on the side of your plate.

Healthy Fat choices:

- ¼ avocado
- ½ T coconut oil
- ½T olive oil
- 1/2-cup Cauliflower Hummus (recipe below)
- 1/8-cup raw seeds (pumpkin or sunflower)
- 14 raw walnut halves
- 20 raw almonds

Sample Dinner:

- 3 ounces of wild caught Salmon seasoned with lemon-pepper seasoning
- 2 cups organic baby greens with ½ T olive oil, cucumbers, peppers and mushrooms
- 1 cup of yellow squash and zucchini cooked in ½ T coconut oil and seasoned with salt, pepper and hot pepper flakes

*Portion size depends on your size. If you have more then 75 lbs. to lose, choose the 4 ounces of protein and have a second afternoon snack; less then 75 lbs., choose the 3 ounces of protein and only choose one afternoon snack.

Evening Snack (Optional): Grain Free Quick Cake

Here you may have a snack if needed. Below is a recipe for a Grain Free Quick Cake made with almond and coconut flour. This cake is low glycemic and is a nice treat at the end of the day.

If you would rather have a snack from the list above, that is fine. Choose just one and only have the evening snack if you are hungry.

Two Weeks of No Alcohol!

If you are a wine or alcohol drinker and having trouble weaning off that evening cocktail, buy some Kombucha and have 8 ounces in a wine glass at night. Kombucha is a fermented tea, which is very good for populating your gut with beneficial bacteria. You will feel like you are having your wine without breaking your detox plan.

Chapter 9: Shopping and Food Preparation

"Processed foods not only extend the shelf life, but they extend the waistline as well."

— Karen Sessions

When cooking your food be sure to use gluten free and chemical free ingredients only. Here is a list of acceptable condiments you may use in your meals.

- Wheat-free tamari
- Mustard
- Sea salt
- Lemons and limes
- Bragg's amino acids
- Bragg's apple cider vinegar
- Bragg's salad dressings
- Seasonings that are free of MSG and "natural" flavors (check your labels)
- Organic coconut oil spray
- Natural leaf stevia or luo han (not Truvia!)
- Coconut oil
- Olive oil

Preparing Foods with Oil

Oils have different smoke points and should be used accordingly. For cooking purposes, Coconut oil is one of the best. It is a saturated fat but it is a medium-chained triglyceride (MCT), which has many health benefits for weight loss, cholesterol reduction and digestive tract health. It has a high smoke point of about 450 degrees so it can safely be heated. Coconut oil has the added benefit of a long lasting shelf life. Be sure to get the virgin organic coconut oil.

Red Palm, Almond, and Avocado oils are also good fats, which are stable at high heat points and make excellent choices for cooking meals.

Best for cold dishes but may be used over a low to medium heat are extra virgin olive oil, walnut oil, sesame oil and peanut oil. Peanut oil must be made from raw, wild peanuts or it will contain aflotoxins, which are carcinogenic. These oils used over a high heat will become unstable, forming free radicals, which can increase your risk of cancer.

When to Choose Organic

Organic refers to the way a crop was grown and processed. To be called organic the plant must be grown in clean soil, have no genetic modifications and not be treated with synthetic pesticides. Natural methods of farming are used to prevent spoilage of the plant by insects and disease. Organic animal products must be free of antibiotics and growth hormone and be free to roam outside and eat an organic diet. Ideally we want to buy as much organic as we can afford.

Each year the Environmental Working Group (EWG) releases a shopping guide of produce with the most and least pesticide residues called The Dirty Dozen and The Clean Fifteen. The vegetables marked organic from the Unlimited Vegetable List are often on this Dirty Dozen guide so I recommend you buy organic for these always. The EWG estimates that if we choose organic for these Dirty Dozen foods we can reduce our intake of pesticides by 80%, which can really make a difference for the toxic load on our bodies.

Coffee and tea as mentioned earlier are also highly sprayed crops and should always be organic.

Organic meats and animal products come from livestock that have not been treated with antibiotics or growth hormones. By choosing organic for your meats, poultry and dairy you are decreasing the toxin load on your body. Again, buy as much organic as you can afford or at the very least choose the leanest animal products as most toxins and hormones are stored in the fatty tissue.

The USDA does not label fish organic so with fish you need to know how to choose clean options. Fish to avoid would be those that are high in mercury or come from an unclean source such as overcrowded farm fisheries. Large fish have higher mercury contents and should be avoided. These would include swordfish, tilefish, marlin, shark, Bluefin tuna and king mackerel. The clean list of fish includes freshwater Coho salmon (US and BC), farmed oysters, wild-caught Pacific sardines, farmed rainbow trout, wild-caught Alaskan salmon, farmed artic char, wild-caught longfin squid (US Atlantic), wild-caught Dungeness crab (CA, OR, WA), farmed mussels, and wild-caught Pacific sardines.

Spices come from crops that may also be heavily sprayed. Organic is always best. Also with spices be sure there are no additives such as MSG or "natural" flavors. Additives found in spices can cause gastrointestinal issues. The word "natural" on a food label has no definition so don't be fooled into thinking it's a healthy food! In fact many hidden harmful ingredients can be disguised under the word natural on the ingredient list of a label.

Buying certified 100% organic food also means you are consuming non-GMO foods. GMO or GM foods (genetically modified organisms or genetically modified) are plants that have had their DNA modified to give them greater resistance to herbicides or improved nutritional content. Some forms of GMO crops are perfectly safe and just meant to cross breed plants to make a better quality food product, however Genetic Engineering or GE crops are a different story and a cause for concern. GE crops are found to be contaminated with high levels of glyphosate due to the fact that they were genetically engineered to withstand high levels of the weed killer, Roundup. Glyphosate has been indicated as a factor in many chronic diseases including but not limited to autism, cancer, obesity, autoimmune disorders and several gastrointestinal diseases such as Crohn's. Glyphosate works to disrupt normal gut bacteria allowing overgrowth of the bad bacteria and killing off the good ones. Corn and soy from the US are almost all GE crops if they are not organic and the by products from these crops are used throughout your processed foods extensively. This is just another good reason to avoid processed foods. Sticking with 100% certified organic foods allows you the peace of mind in knowing you are not ingesting any GE foods that may inflict harm on your health.

An easy way to tell how your produce was grown is to look at the produce code on the sticker of the fruit or vegetable. A four digit code beginning with the number 4 means it was conventionally grown, a 5-digit code beginning with the number 9 means it was organically grown and a 5-digit code beginning with the number 8 means it was genetically modified.

Easy Vegetable Wash to Remove Pesticides

Not everyone can always afford organic and even so there may still be some pesticide residue on the fruits and vegetables. We can't avoid what's already been absorbed into the skins but getting the surface as clean as possible can get rid of a large percentage of the pesticides. In addition, this wash will help preserve your produce so it lasts longer without spoiling.

In a large bowl put 3 parts water to 1 part white vinegar. Let the fruits and vegetables soak for 30 minutes to 1 hour. Rinse, dry and store until ready to eat.

Chapter 10: Recipes

"This is my advice to people: Learn how to cook, try new recipes, learn from your mistakes, be fearless, and above all have fun."

— Julia Child

Mary's Detox Soup

- 1 T coconut oil
- 1 medium sweet onion, chopped
- 2 garlic cloves, minced
- 8 stalks of organic celery, chopped
- 1 leek, chopped
- 1 medium rutabaga, peeled and chopped
- 5 organic tomatoes, chopped (3 cups) or 1 box POMI chopped tomatoes
- 8 cups of organic, unsalted vegetable or chicken stock
- 4 cups of fresh, chopped, organic kale
- Salt and pepper to taste (I use about ½ tsp. of each)

In a large stock pan heat the coconut oil over medium heat.

Add onions, garlic, and leek and cook for about 3-4 minutes.

Add rutabaga and celery and cook for an additional 5 minutes.

Add the tomatoes and the unsalted stock, bring to a simmer and cover for 15 minutes or until rutabaga is soft.

When the soup is done, remove from heat and add the kale and cover the pot to allow kale to cook for a few minutes in the hot soup. Soup may be very thick so be prepared to add additional water to thin it out.

Add salt and pepper to taste.

This recipe makes a lot of soup, so freeze half of it for your second week.

Crock Pot option: Place all ingredients in pot and cook on high for 6 hours.

Cauliflower Hummus

- 1 T coconut or olive oil
- 1 16oz. bag of riced cauliflower
- 2 garlic cloves, peeled and minced
- 1 tsp. cumin
- ½ tsp. pepper
- ½ tsp. salt
- 3 T tahini
- juice from ½ lemon (I love Meyers lemons)

Heat oil over medium in a saucepan. Add garlic and cauliflower, stirring frequently until slightly browned.

Add spices and cook 1 minute. Transfer to a high-speed blender and add tahini and lemon juice. Mix until blended.

Serving size: ¼ cup

Makes about 9 servings

Grain Free Quick Cake

- 1 T almond flour
- 2 tsp. coconut flour
- 1/2 tsp. baking powder
- 1 pack stevia
- ¼ cup egg whites
- 1 T pumpkin or applesauce
- 1 tsp. unsweetened cocoa or carob

In a microwave safe ramekin or mug, mix all the dry ingredients first. Add egg whites and stir well until ingredients are all blended.

Microwave for 1 minute (time may vary). If you saved your berries from the morning shake you can add them to the cake and cook it a bit longer (about 15-30 extra seconds).

Chia Seed Milkshake

- 1 cup unsweetened almond or coconut milk
- 1 T chia seeds (soaked in the milk 15-20 minutes)
- 1 tsp. cocoa or carob
- 1 packet stevia
- 5-6 ice cubes

Place milk and chia seeds in the blender and let it sit for at least 15 minutes. Add all other ingredients to the blender and mix until thick and creamy. Enjoy this amazing, healthy, low glycemic snack with no guilt.

Look for more recipes in BodyDesigns Detox Friendly Recipes Book available in e-book when you purchase this plan. Please contact me for a copy if you did not receive one.

Chapter 11: Challenging Foods

"Insanity is doing the same thing
over and over again and expecting different results."
—Albert Einstein (attributed)

The Detox Plan is meant to change your lifestyle. Going back to old eating habits will make you fat and sick again. Staying off of processed foods and limiting carbohydrates, especially from sugar, will be an important strategy moving forward to keep the weight off and stay healthy. Some people will find that gluten and/or dairy were the cause of some health issues so it's important to do a trial of each of these foods after the Detox is finished. First, introduce dairy into your diet once or twice a day for 1-3 days. Make sure it's in a pure form and doesn't contain sugar and other additives so you can determine if it is truly the dairy that poses a problem. Look for signs of gastrointestinal distress, inflammation, headaches, rashes, depression, weight gain, etc. If you have any symptoms, stop the dairy immediately. If not, you can continue to enjoy organic dairy in your new lifestyle plan.

Next, add back gluten at least twice a day for 1-3 days. Again, make sure your source is very clean and doesn't contain other chemicals and preservatives that may affect how you feel. Ezekiel bread might be a good choice. If dairy was an issue, make sure there is no dairy in the product. If gluten does not seem to bother you, then you may begin to have it in your new lifestyle plan. However, keep in mind just because it is gluten free does not mean it can be used in abundance in any lifestyle diet plan because it is still found in high carbohydrate foods that spike insulin.

If you wish to continue with your weight loss or need help with a lifestyle diet plan, please contact BodyDesigns for a Personalized Diet Plan. With a Personalized Diet Plan you get specific meal and snack choices throughout the day all individualized to your likes, dislikes, and goals. All clients receive a phone or Skype consultation, a personalized diet plan by email, full access to an array of clean and easy recipes, and support for a month with daily monitoring of food logs. For more information visit **BodyDesignsbyMary.com** and click on the Nutrition tab.

Appendix 1:
Unlimited Vegetable List

- Artichokes/hearts
- Asparagus
- Bamboo shoots
- Bean sprouts
- Broccoli
- Brussels sprouts
- Cabbage
- Carrots (1/2 cup)
- Cauliflower
- Celery (organic)
- Cucumber (organic)
- Eggplant
- Green beans
- Greens – kale, spinach, all greens (organic)
- Leeks
- Mushrooms
- Okra
- Onions
- Peppers (organic)
- Radishes
- Salad greens (organic)
- Sugar snap peas (imported, organic)
- Summer squash (organic)
- Swiss chard
- Tomatoes (organic)
- Turnips
- Water chestnuts
- Zucchini

Appendix 2: Shopping List

Copy this list and check off the items you will need for your detox plan. You won't need everything on this list so don't just go out and buy it all. Take the time to plan out your meals and snacks then check off the foods you need to buy. In Appendix 3 you will find suggestions on where you might find some of the items.

___Lemons or organic lemon juice

___Bragg's apple cider vinegar

___Natural leaf stevia (see Appendix 3)

___Organic coffee

___Organic tea

___Teeccino

___Unsweetened Vanilla or Plain Almond Milk (see Appendix 3)

___Unsweetened Vanilla or Plain Coconut Milk (see Appendix 3)

___Unsweetened Vanilla or Plain Cashew Milk (see Appendix 3)

___Vegan Protein Shake (see Appendix 3)

___Spirulina (see Appendix 3)

___Chia Seeds (see Appendix 3)

BodyDesigns Two-Week Detox Plan

___Bananas

___Avocados

___Organic berries (frozen are fine)

___Organic chicken

___Grass fed beef

___Wild Alaskan Salmon (canned is fine, try to find PBA free cans)

___Organic tofu

___Organic Tempeh

___Organic eggs

___Organic greens for salads

___Tahini

___Coconut oil (see Appendix 3)

___Olive oil

___Raw nuts

___Raw pumpkin seeds

___Raw sunflower seeds

___Almond butter

___Cashew butter

___Bragg's amino acids (see Appendix 3)

___Bragg's salad dressing (see Appendix 3)

___Kombucha

___Vegetables from Unlimited Vegetable List

_____

_____

_____

_____

_____

_____

_____

_____

_____

_____

Ingredients for Detox soup

___coconut oil

___sweet onion

___leek

___celery

___garlic cloves

___tomatoes or POMI carton of tomatoes

___unsalted stock

___organic kale

___medium rutabaga

Ingredients for Cauliflower Hummus

___1-16 oz. package riced cauliflower

___tahini

___garlic

___cumin

___salt

___lemon

___pepper

Ingredients for Grain Free Quick Cake

___almond flour

___coconut flour

___baking powder

___egg whites

___unsweetened carob or unsweetened cocoa

Appendix 3: Product Guide

Vegan Protein – my favorite is Sunwarrior Raw Blend (not original). This can be found at The Vitamin Shoppe, Sprouts, Earthfare, Amazon.com or at Sunwarrior.com

Bragg's makes so many good products. Bragg's amino acids are a gluten free substitute for soy sauce and you might like it in your cooking. Bragg's also makes great salad dressings that are gluten free and of course they are famous for their apple cider vinegar. You can usually find Bragg's products in the health food section of your grocery store, Whole Foods, Sprouts, Earthfare or online.

Teeccino as mentioned above is an herbal coffee substitute. It can be found in local health food stores, Sprouts, Whole Foods or online at Amazon.com.

Unsweetened Almond, Cashew or Coconut Milk should not contain carrageenan. Try Silk, Trader Joes or Whole Foods 365 for almond milk or Cashew and So Delicious or Native Forest for coconut milk.

Spirulina powder (not capsule) is found in the supplement section of your health food store or online at Amazon.com. Make sure it's organic or use Nutrex Hawaiian brand.

Chia Seeds are usually found in a grocery store health food section, Costco, The Vitamin Shop or online at Amazon.com.

Coconut oil must be virgin and organic and can be found in most stores. Costco sells a large container at a great price. Coconut oil will last for years so don't be afraid to buy the large one.

Stevia must be a natural leaf without any additives. Look for NOW organic stevia or Sweet Leaf for your best choices. Monk fruit is also an excellent sweetener.

Kombucha is fermented tea and can be found at Whole Foods and many grocery and natural food stores throughout the country. This refreshing beverage is low in sugar and beneficial for gut health.

For a Getting Started Guide listing more product information please contact me and I will be happy to send you one. I can be reached at BodyDesignsbyMary.com.

About the Author

Mary graduated from the University of Delaware with a degree in Nutrition and Dietetics. She continued her education receiving a Masters degree in Nutrition from Rutgers University and becoming a Registered Dietitian. She has developed and implemented wellness and weight loss programs for the University of Medicine and Dentistry of New Jersey while serving as a faculty member in the residency program. As a consultant, she has worked in various weight loss programs including Scottish Rite's Shapedown for children.

She is certified in personal training by the American Council of Exercise (ACE) and currently owns and manages BodyDesigns. BodyDesigns offers personalized diets, nutrition coaching and exercise programs that help people transform their lifestyles for weight loss and optimal wellness

Sources and References

Beck, Leslie. "The Safest Fish to Eat? Follow This Rule, New Study Suggests." *The Globe and Mail*. N.p., 7 Aug. 2012. Web. 12 Oct. 2014. <http://www.theglobeandmail.com/life/health-and-fitness/health/the-safest-fish-to-eat-follow-this-rule-new-study-suggests/article4467061/>.

Carr, Kris. "How to Maintain PH Balance in the Body | Acidic vs. Alkaline Foods." *KrisCarrcom RSS*. Kris Carr, 2 Sept. 2014. Web. 12 Oct. 2014. <http://kriscarr.com/blog-video/ph-balance-alkaline-foods/>.

"Chattering Kitchen." *Chattering Kitchen*. N.p., n.d. Web. 11 Oct. 2014. <http://chatteringkitchen.com/culinary-quotes/>.

Coles, Terri. "10 Reasons To Add Chia To Your Diet." *The Huffington Post*. N.p., 3 June 2013. Web. 12 Oct. 2014. <http://www.huffingtonpost.ca/2013/06/03/chia-seed-benefits-_n_3379831.html>.

Colquhoun, James. "The 6 Greatest Cholesterol Myths Debunked." *Food Matters*. JAMES COLQUHOUN, 10 Sept. 2014. Web. 10 Sept. 2014. <http://foodmatters.tv/articles-1/the-6-greatest-cholesterol-myths-debunked>.

"Dr. Swanson: GMOs Cause Increase in Chronic Diseases, Infertility and Birth Defects." *Sustainable Pulse*. N.p., 27 Apr. 2013. Web. 12 Oct. 2014.

<http://sustainablepulse.com/2013/04/27/dr-swanson-gmos-and-roundup-increase-chronic-diseases-infertility-and-birth-defects/#.VDb6CCldUg5>.

Endelman, Rob. "The Delicious Truth: The Difference Between the Terms "GE" and "GMO"" *The Delicious Truth: The Difference Between the Terms "GE" and "GMO"* N.p., 23 Mar. 2012. Web. 10 Oct. 2014. <http://thedelicioustruth.blogspot.com/2012/03/difference-between-terms-ge-and-gmo.html>.

Gottfired, Sara. "How To Get A Grip On Food If You're An Overeater." *MindBodyGreen*. N.p., 13 Sept. 2014. Web. 12 Oct. 2014. <http://www.mindbodygreen.com/0-15276/how-to-get-a-grip-on-food-if-youre-an-overeater.html>.

Hawkins, Amanda. "Your Guide to Shopping the Produce Aisle." *Good Housekeeping*. N.p., n.d. Web. 12 Oct. 2014.

<http://www.goodhousekeeping.com/health/nutrition/fruits-and-vegetables-to-buy-organic>.

"Health Quotes." *Detox My Day*. N.p., n.d. Web. 12 Oct. 2014.
<http://detoxmyday.wordpress.com/health-quotes/>.

"Hippocrates Quotes." *Hippocrates Quotes (Author of Hippocratic Writings)*. N.p., n.d. Web. 12 Oct. 2014.
<https://www.goodreads.com/author/quotes/248774.Hippocrates>.

"Hormone." *MedicineNet*. N.p., 19 Mar. 2012. Web. 09 Oct. 2014.
<http://www.medterms.com/script/main/art.asp?articlekey=3783>.

"How to Lose Weight with a Fatty Liver." *Liver Doctor*. N.p., n.d. Web. 12 Oct. 2014. <http://www.liverdoctor.com/how-to-lose-weight-with-a-fatty-liver/>.

Hyman, Mark. "Fat Doesn't Not Make You Fat." *DrMarkHyman.com*. Dr. Mark Hyman, 27 Nov. 2013. Web. <http:// drhyman.com/blog/2013/11/26/fat-make-fat/ >.

Hyman, Mark. "Frankenfoods » Issues » Explore More: Genetic Engineering." *Frankenfoods » Issues » Explore More: Genetic Engineering*. N.p., n.d. Web. 12 Oct. 2014. <http://www.iptv.org/exploremore/ge/issues/issue4.cfm>.

Hyman, Mark. "Why Did Saturated Fat Get a Bad Rep? *Dr. Mark Hyman*. N.p., 8 Sept. 2014. Web. 12 Oct. 2014.
<http://drhyman.com/blog/2014/09/08/saturated-fat-get-bad-rep/>

Hyman, Mark. "Are You Also Being Deceived into Eating Fake Frankenfoods?." *Dr. Mark Hyman*. N.p., 15 Nov. 2012. Web. 12 Oct. 2014.

<http://drhyman.com/blog/2010/07/04/are-you-also-being-deceived-into-eating-fake-frankenfoods/>

"Jasper Carrott Quote." *BrainyQuote*. Xplore, n.d. Web. 12 Oct. 2014.
<http://www.brainyquote.com/quotes/quotes/j/jaspercarr281919.html>.

Johnson, J. L., D. S. Duick, and S. A. Aldasouqi. "Identifying Prediabetes Using Fasting Insulin Levels." *National Center for Biotechnology Information*. U.S. National Library of Medicine, Jan. 2010. Web. 12 Oct. 2014.
<http://www.ncbi.nlm.nih.gov/pubmed/19789156>.

Layton, Julia. "Is Lack of Sleep Making Me Fat?" *HowStuffWorks.* HowStuffWorks.com, 6 Oct. 2008. Web. 12 Oct. 2014. <http://science.howstuffworks.com/life/sleep-obesity1.htm>.

"Mark Twain Quote." *BrainyQuote.* Xplore, n.d. Web. 12 Oct. 2014. <http://www.brainyquote.com/quotes/quotes/m/marktwain118964.html>.

Meara, Clair O. "Spirulina Powder Review." *Spirulina Powder Review.* N.p., 5 Jan. 2014. Web. 12 Oct. 2014. <http://spirulinapowder-review.com/>.

Mercola, Dr. "Sugar Substitutes: What's Safe and What's Not?" *Mercola.com.* N.p., 7 Oct. 2013. Web. 12 Oct. 2014. <http://articles.mercola.com/sites/articles/archive/2013/10/07/sugar-substitutes.aspx>.

"Organic Foods: What You Need to Know." *Health Education.* Familydoctor.org, Sept. 2011. Web. 12 Oct. 2014. <http://familydoctor.org/familydoctor/en/prevention-wellness/food-nutrition/healthy-food-choices/organic-foods-what-you-need-to-know.html>.

"Paper, Research, and Special Focus Meeting Report. Current Level of Consensus on Probiotic Science (n.d.): N. Pag. Current Level of Consensus on Probiotic Science. Ian Rowland,1,* Lucio Capurso,2 Kevin Collins,3 John Cummings,4 Nathalie Delzenne,5 Olivier Goulet,6 Francisco Guarner,7 Philippe Marteau8 and Rémy Meier9, Nov. 2010. Web. ." . N.p., n.d. Web. 12 Nov. 2010. <http://www.landesbioscience.com/journals/gutmicrobes/RowlandGMIC1-6.pdf>.

"Quotations by Author." *Albert Einstein Quotes.* N.p., n.d. Web. 12 Oct. 2014. <http://www.quotationspage.com/quotes/Albert_Einstein/41>.

"Quotes About Food." *(1293 Quotes).* N.p., n.d. Web. 12 Oct. 2014. <https://www.goodreads.com/quotes/tag/food?page=3>.

Samsel, Anthony, and Stephanie Seneff. "Glyphosate's Suppression of Cytochrome P450 Enzymes and Amino Acid Biosynthesis by the Gut Microbiome: Pathways to Modern Diseases†." *Entropy.* N.p., 10 Apr. 2013. Web. 12 Oct. 2014. <http://www.mdpi.com/1099-4300/15/4/1416>.

Story, Colleen M. "What's the Best Oil to Cook With?" *Renegade Health*. N.p., 28 Aug. 2013. Web. 12 Oct. 2014. <http://renegadehealth.com/blog/2013/08/28/whats-the-best-oil-to-cook-with>.

Trimarchi, Maria. "How Organic Farming Works." *HowStuffWorks*. HowStuffWorks.com, 18 Dec. 2007. Web. 12 Oct. 2014. <http://science.howstuffworks.com/environmental/green-science/organic-farming2.htm>.

"Vegetable Broth." *The Dr. Oz Show*. N.p., 19 Mar. 2014. Web. 12 Oct. 2014. <http://www.doctoroz.com/recipe/dr-ozs-2-week-rapid-weight-loss-plan-vegetable-broth>.

Walton, Alice G. "How Much Sugar Are Americans Eating? [Infographic]." *Forbes*. Forbes Magazine, 30 Aug. 2012. Web. 12 Oct. 2014. <http://www.forbes.com/sites/alicegwalton/2012/08/30/how-much-sugar-are-americans-eating-infographic/>.

"Western Pattern Diet." *Wikipedia*. Wikimedia Foundation, 10 Dec. 2014. Web. 12 Oct. 2014. <http://en.wikipedia.org/wiki/Western_pattern_diet>.

Thank You
for Reading

Please take a moment to
share your thoughts and reactions

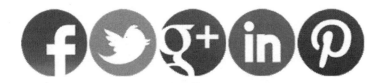

Read on GoodReads.com

Made in the USA
Columbia, SC
18 June 2020

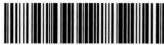